Methods of Birth Control

Other books by Lewis Warsh:

The Suicide Rates
Highjacking
Moving Through Air
Dreaming As One
Long Distance
Part of My History
Immediate Surrounding
Today
The Maharajah's Son
Blue Heaven
Hives

Methods of Birth Control
By Lewis Warsh

Sun & Moon Press
Washington, D.C. and *Philadelphia*

©Lewis Warsh, 1983

All rights reserved. Except for brief passages quoted in newspaper, magazine, radio, or television reviews, no part of this publication may be published, reproduced, read publicly, distributed or transmitted, in any forms or media, or by any other means, electronic or mechanical, including photocopy, recording, or any information storage and retrieval system now known or to be invented, without permission in writing from the author, his authorized agent(s), or his heirs.

ISBN: 0-940650-21-5
First Edition
Library of Congress Catalog Card Number: 83-060975

Sun & Moon Press Contemporary Literature Series no. 16
Sun & Moon: A Journal of Literature & Art, no. 13

Grateful acknowledgement is made to *United Artists* magazine in which ''Eye Opener,'' ''The Genetic Ode'' and ''Methods of Birth Control'' first appeared.

cover drawing: Rackstraw Downes

Publication of this book has been made possible, in part, through matching grants from The National Endowment for the Arts and The Maryland Arts Council.

Sun & Moon Press
4330 Hartwick Road
College Park, Maryland 20740

for Peggy DeCoursey

Eye Opener

I

Light rays which pass
through the transparent media of the eye
are focused on the macula
when the eye is at rest

II

Detailed vision is the result of
the projection of an image
on the specialized portion
of the retina known as the macula

III

When the optic nerve enters the eye
there is no overlying retina

IV

In the nerve-head
light cannot be translated
into nerve impulses

V

Test cards for color vision
have been constructed with a
background of carefully printed
and selected colored dots into
which have been blended
dots of a contrasting shade
to form numerals

VI

The color-blind person is confused
by the colors and shades

VII

Distinguish the number or see it
as a different number

VIII

A person wearing glasses is no longer conspicuous
unless he chooses decorative frames,
by preference

IX

One out of every four children needs glasses

X

If involved with tasks dangerous to your eyes
wear safety goggles

XI

An eye may turn in,
roll up or down
or swing out

XII

Jews have more nearsightedness (myopia)
than Blacks in whom farsightedness
(hyperopia) is predominant

XIII

One hears parents urging children to keep
their glasses on

XIV

Various cultists have offered hope
that exercise will relieve the need
for glasses

XV

The earliest known lens was found
in the ruins of Nineveh, Assyria

XVI

The origin of glass is lost in antiquity

XVII

The crucible in which optical glass
is made is of clay aged
for three months under rigidly
controlled conditions

XVIII

Accented bifocals were devised
with a supplementary lens glued
with Canada balsam to the one
for distance correction

XIX

A flowing depression is ground
into a crown glass distance blank

XX

In China, tortoise-shell frames
were worn without lenses
as a sign of dignity

XXI

It was a simple step from Bacon's
magnifying glass laid on the page
to get a lens in a frame which
could be held in the hand

XXII

Lorgnettes are generally used
for rapid reference only

XXIII

Prismatic spectacles are useful
to persons who have diseases
which make it necessary for them
to remain in the supine position

XXIV

Pliny recorded that Nero wore a colored lens
attached to his thumb

XXV

Dark lenses manufactured as prescription
glasses may have bifocal segments
if desired

XXVI

Opticians are technicians

skilled in the making
of spectacles

XXVII

Farsighted eyes are smaller
than the normal eye
by a fraction of an inch in
the distance from cornea to
retina

XXVIII

The lens is dislocated backwards
towards the vitreous

XXIX

A retina which has not been
adequately stimulated
must learn to see

XXX

When we are ill
or out of sorts
no part of our bodies functions
as well as when we are well
and full of energy

XXXI

Children suffering from hyperopia

who cannot describe their trouble
discover that when they look out
the window their difficulty is eased
and they become happier

XXXII

Nearsighted people do not know what they do not see

XXXIII

Objects do not appear blurred to everyone

XXXIV

Some of these eyes will turn out

XXXV

Progressive myopia is characterized
by a family history of its occurrence

XXXVI

A severely nearsighted person
shouldn't undertake exercises
or sports in which his head
may receive sharp blows, such as
boxing or high diving

XXXVII

Since myopia was first known
people have speculated as to
its cause

XXXVIII

Progressive myopia is thought
to be passed on according
to the laws of the inheritance
of recessive characters
as described by Mendel

XXXIX

The nearsighted person no longer need
feel unusual because
he's wearing glasses

XL

When an object is viewed
it will be evenly out of focus
because it is focused
in front of or in back of
the receptive tissue known as the macula

XLI

Changes in the lens of the eye,
i.e. a cataract, can bend light rays
irrationally

XLII

One meridian is myopic,
another is hyperopic

XLIII

There are no known sexual differences
in the incidence of astigmatism

XLIV

Myopia, myopia
with astigmatism,
myopic astigmatism

total myopia

XLV

Most babies are born with corneal astigmatism

XLVI

A patient surveying a newly
placed drapery remarked that the
horizontally striped material

used on the valence was not of
the same bolt of cloth as that
of the vertically hanging side pieces

XLVII

Headaches located in the front of the head
or over the whole head

XLVIII

The head may be held
at an angle
to compensate
for the blurred
image

XLIX

Neck muscles may be treated
as the cause of tilted heads

L

The optician proceeds to manufacture the required lens

LI

The Romans dealt with the poor
near vision of old age by getting
young slaves to read to them

LII

A short person with short arms
will need reading glasses sooner
than a tall person

LIII

It's highly desirable that a
complete medical eye-examination
be done at this time

LIV

Time was when people
had to have reading glasses,
plus another pair of glasses,
for correction of distance vision

LV

It may be necessary to perform
an operation known as
dacryocystorhinostomy

LVI

The conjunctival lining
of the eyelid is known as
the palpebral conjunctiva,
that of the eyeball
the bulbar conjunctiva

LVII

Usually colobomas are small and inconspicuous

LVIII

A notch in the lid margin
in which there is no skin and lashes

LIX

An extra row of eyelashes
where the glands open into the
lid margins

LX

The muscles which move the eye are
attached at their posterior ends
to a ring in the back of an orbit,
the annule of Zinn

LXI

A glistening white tissue which
blends into the cornea at the limbus

LXII

Corneal lenses afloat on a film of tears

LXIII

A small foreign body may be washed away
by the tears

LXIV

Eyes fixed with corrective lenses
tend to grow progressively weaker
and to require progressively stronger
lenses for their correction

LXV

If crippled eyes could be
transformed into crippled legs
every other person would go limping
by

LXVI

The palliation of symptoms
is not the only treatment
for defective vision

LXVII

Petty adventurers and charlatans
hang upon the skirts of society
ever ready and eager to take
advantage of human suffering

LXVIII

The unwarranted assumption that
the whole business is mere quackery
is widely accepted

LXIX

Licensed charlatanism among
opticians has been described
and denounced in articles appearing
in *The Readers Digest* and
The New York World-Telegram

LXX

As long as the organs of vision
are used under a condition of
mental and physical tension
the visual defects will persist
or actually become worse

LXXI

Occasionally nature effects a
spontaneous cure, and the old
habits of seeing are restored
instantaneously

LXXII

Her vision was so improved that
she immediately picked up a telephone
book and read it

LXXIII

Rest the tips of your fingers
upon a table and the contact
at the end of a few minutes
will no longer be felt

LXXIV

The intensity of the light falling
upon the page of your book will be
in the neighborhood of ten thousand
foot-candles

LXXV

Ten feet away from the window
the illumination may fall to
two foot-candles

LXXVI

People with relaxed organs of
vision find their sense-field
filled with blackness

LXXVII

One thousand foot-candles in the shade of a tree

LXXVIII

In the case of long-sighted persons,
especially those having a tendency
to squint, nervous tension is often
extreme

LXXIX

The intensification of the disturbance
increases the dysfunction and so
heightens the tension

LXXX

Mal-functioning and strain
tend to appear
whenever the conscious "I"
interferes with instinctively
acquired habits of use

LXXXI

The conscious "I" interferes
with the process of seeing
even at times when no
emotional distresses are present

LXXXII

Clear seeing is the result of
accurate sensing and correct perceiving

LXXXIII

Any improvement in the power of
perceiving tends to be accompanied
by an improvement in the power
of sensing and of that product of
sensing and perceiving which is seeing

LXXXIV

The eye without errors of refraction
cannot see clearly through a lens
designed to correct an error
it no longer has

LXXXV

An eye cannot see clearly through a lens

The Genetic Ode

I

Genetically uniform races arrive through forms
of uniparental reproduction

II

An individual heterozygous for 31 pairs of genes
could produce more than 2 billion
kinds of spermatozoa with different complements

III

In the Malay-Indonesian
languages the word *keturunan*
stands for biological
inheritance, *warisan*
for inheritance of property

IV

Some people are born clever, others stupid

V

Erect posture
ability to subsist on diverse diets
absence of a breeding system

VI

In Muller's utopia it might
be possible to perpetuate a mankind
consisting only of mules

VII

Barring mutation, nobody can transmit
to his descendants any genes
other than those which
he himself has received

VIII

The hereditary materials in sex cells
are arrays of discrete units

IX

Gemmules lodged in sex cells expand
to form the body of the next generation

X

The gemmules were supposed to originate in the body cells

XI

When the sex cells give
rise to an embryo, the *gemmules*
(as Darwin called them) become
transformed into new body cells
of the type that formed them
originally

XII

Leeuwenhoeck saw within the spermatozoon
a miniature likeness of the human body

XIII

A taste for good wines is passed on to his progeny

XIV

Material comforts come to almost everybody
at least to those capable of wanting and appreciating
them

XV

Banks of corneas can be kept ready to be transplanted
to damaged eyes

XVI

The surgeon transfers to the
appropriate place a piece of
skin taken from the patient's
thigh

XVII

A prick on the skin
of the leg may cause
a reflex motion of the leg

XVIII

The individual may be thin, hyperexcitable
and suffer from insomnia

XIX

If a large piece of the liver
is removed from an adult
rat, the liver cells
which had stopped dividing when
the liver reached the adult
size, start dividing again

XX

A brain, a liver, a heart
4 limbs

XXI

From the humblest seaweed
to the giant forest trees

XXII

The insulin molecule becomes
active only after a pair of
enzymes cut off a stretch of
33 amino acids from the middle
of the chain

XXIII

Enzymes concentrated
in cellular particles
called mitochondria

XXIV

The flight muscles of birds
use oxygen from blood
to oxidize sugar

XXV

Blood carries lactic acid to the liver for disposal

XXVI

Genes are judged by the level
at which their protein
products function

XXVII

Altered genes increase
the reproductive performance
of the organism

natural selection

XXVIII

An increase in temperature increases the number
of collisions

XXIX

Adenosine triphosphate
can act as a donor
to a phosphate group

XXX

The rigid structure of bone
is a product of the chemical
activity of bone cells
which are embedded in the bone
and build and rebuild all the time

XXXI

An increase in disorder means some energy has been dissipated

XXXII

All eggs are present
at birth and mature one
a month after puberty

XXXIII

A cell of a given
type in man resembles
an analogous cell in
a fish or a frog or
a fly more than
it resembles a cell
from a different
human organ

XXXIV

Fish in underground lakes lose their eyelids

XXXV

In time the bacteria would become mitochondria

XXXVI

Cells of an evolving line, possibly
amoebalike, unable to use oxygen, may
have ingested bacteria

XXXVII

Cells that use a great deal of
energy very fast, such as the flight
muscles of birds, have enormous amounts
of mitochondria

XXXVIII

All eucaryotic cells contain some
membrane-enveloped vesicles, the mitochondria

XXXIX

No nuclear membrane, no chromosomes, no mitosis

XL

The outer layer of the cell
is a double layer of fatty
molecules

XLI

A particle of polio virus
is simply a piece of nucleic
acid

XLII

Hereditary messages of genes
are translated into structures
of protein

XLIII

Transcription of DNA
to make messenger RNA
is done by an enzyme

RNA polymearse

XLIV

From the sequence of nucleotides
to the sequence of amino acids

XLV

Xeroderma pigmentosum
is caused by a genetic defect
in a DNA repairing system

XLVI

Information represented in the
sequence of molecules

XLVII

The principle of complementary pairing
between sequences of nucleic acid
bases is the only mechanism available
for the specific transfer
of information

XLVIII

A base, a sugar
phosphate

XLIX

Proteins, amino acids
nucleic acids, nucleotides

L

Different amino acids are ordered
in different sequences
in different proteins

LI

The gene acts as a template

LII

The cellulose of plants
is a repetitive polymer
consisting of chains of
identical glucose monomers
successively linked to
one another in the same way

LIII

Polymers in which monomers
are joined together
in a linear sequence

LIV

Genes from different chromosomes come together
and exchange parts

LV

Amoebae or bacteria
produce copies of themselves by
simple fission

LVI

Unique cranial capacity

LVII

Half the sperms receive an X
chromosome and when they join
an egg gives rise to XX pairs

LVIII

Unconfirmed reports say
XYY may be prone to violence

LIX

Occasionally man is born with one X and 2 Ys

LX

A lottery of innumerable combinations
of genes in the egg and the sperm

LXI

Mixed blood

pure blood

LXII

The lottery takes place that decides in
random fashion which copy of a gene
a sperm or egg gets

LXIII

The orderly transmission from parents to
offspring of elements which remain
unchanged

LXIV

Inbred brown rabbits have two copies of a "brown" gene

LXV

Two identical parents generate identical progeny

LXVI

Inbred lines of animals
can be created
by repeated
brother-to-sister
matings in
rats, mice
and rabbits

LXVII

Flowering plants depend on wind or
often insect visitors to bring together
sperm and egg

LXVIII

Continuity of evolution through the passing self

LXIX

Each parent

High Fidelity

I

Big loudspeakers for low-frequency reproduction
are not only inefficient but full of distortion

II

The bigger the traducer, the greater
the distortion

III

The phonograph pickup is a traducer

IV

Microphones, phonograph
cartridges, loudspeakers

V

A loudspeaker is a traducer which
converts variations in electrical
energy into the mechanical, in-
and-out motion of a cone or diaphragm

VI

The wiggles of the stylus in the groove
are converted into variations
of electrical energy

VII

Resistance-coupled amplifiers
become available through some of
the jobbers as ready-wired units

VIII

The voice coil moves in and out of

a cylindrical slot in the magnet
structure

IX

Electricity generated by the amplifier
forces the cone through a cycle of motion

X

From an at-rest position, outward,
back past the at-rest position
to a negative or "withdrawn"
position, and back to rest again

XI

Pre World War II type loudspeakers
did not use permanent magnets

XII

The more precise the relationship
between voice coil and magnet,
the greater the tolerances

XIII

If the cone is allowed to
ride free around the outer edge
it would eventually pull the voice
coil into contact with the magnet

XIV

A centering device at the apex
of the cone, near the voice coil

XV

To maintain the sound level the
sound of the cone and/or

the distance it travels
must be increased

XVI

The effective diameter of the cone
would have to be doubled or the distance
it travelled would have to be
quadrupled

XVII

The bigger the cone
the narrower the beam

XVIII

For the chair position
the loss of highs
would become noticeable
above 2,500 cycles

XIX

The result of cone breakup is ragged response
at high frequencies

XX

Some speakers have diffusers near the voice-coil area

XXI

The sound hits the wall and bounces back into the room

XXII

Aim the speaker at the ceiling

XXIII

The resonant frequency approaches the cone-breakup
frequency

XXIV

How rapidly the resonant
frequency drops depends
on the size of the baffle

XXV

Factors such as enclosure
design and amplifier design
are normally adjusted to
reduce the hump

XXVI

If the baffle is small
the attenuation rate will
be about 18 db per octave

XXVII

The voice coil is no longer centered in the magnet gap

XXVIII

When the electricity is cut off,
the coil (and the cone) will snap back

XXIX

A bigger cone is more difficult
to control or damp

XXX

If a stiff-suspension system
is used to help damping,
cone resonance rises

XXXI

If you have ample room,
use a big woofer
and a tweeter

XXXII

A large-cone speaker emits sound
in a beam which narrows rapidly
as the frequency increases

XXXIII

A coaxial speaker has *two* voice coils operating around
the same axis

XXXIV

One cone for the woofer
one diaphragm for the tweeter

XXXV

A direct-radiator speaker
opens directly out of the
baffle

XXXVI

A loudspeaker mounted as a direct-radiator
in a large, flat baffle

XXXVII

Pulsations of the cone force the air out
sideways

XXXVIII

A 15-watt speaker could
handle a transient peak
of 30 watts

XXXIX

Tap the cone to estimate cone-resonance frequency

XL

A wire resists the flow of
electricity, and the amount
of resistance is measured
in ohms

XLI

Resistance varies with the frequency
of the alternating current

XLII

Impedance is the alternating current synonym
for resistance

XLIII

The speaker isn't mounted in any sort of baffle

XLIV

Most speakers have a nominal voice-coil
impedance of 16 ohms

XLV

Frequency response
harmonic distortion
intermodulation distortion
noise and hum level

XLVI

Watts output
input level
gain
input impedance
output impedance
damping factor

XLVII

Harmonic distortion in an amplifier
is determined by measuring the strength
of the original frequency

XLVIII

At 10 watts output the amplifier
is said to have 1 percent
harmonic distortion

XLIX

In a manner similar to that
used for harmonic distortion
measurements, the original signals
are removed and the strength
of the spurious frequencies
are measured and stated as a
percentage of the voltage
of the original frequencies

L

The loudness of regular sound
when the amplifier is turned on full

LI

Apply ''square'' waves to the input
and check the output with an oscilloscope

LII

Square wave pictures demonstrate transient response

LIII

Room resonances increase the apparent loudness
of low frequencies

LIV

Boosting the base through tone-control adjustment
cannot be considered a solution to speaker inefficiency

LV

Gain is the amount of amplification
provided by an amplifier

LVI

A mismatch between amplifier and speaker
may result in distortion

LVII

Some heavy-feedback amplifiers
oscillate i.e. motorboat
under conditions not foreseen
when they were designed

LVIII

Loudness and volume are controlled by the same knob

LIX

In some units two separate knobs,
mounted concentrically, are provided

LX

The range of loudness compensation
will depend on the position
of the loudness switch

LXI

Bass tone control increases (''boosts'')
or decreases (''cuts'') low frequencies progressively
as the frequency decreases

LXII

The turnover point is the same
for A and B, but A holds back
its effect whereas B will produce
a noticeable cut

LXIII

If the control unit does
not incorporate a loudness
control, the bass tone control
can be used to make up
for apparent low-frequency
deficiencies when the volume is
turned down

LXIV

Nearly all control units
include one or two knobs

LXV

A single multiposition knob
is used to combine bass and
treble in one control

LXVI

Equalization knobs could be eliminated
leaving minor adjustments to tone controls

LXVII

Bass boost may be achieved
by boosting the amplitude of the
low-frequency signals, but it is
more often done by depressing
the middles and highs

LXVIII

Fixed preamps incorporate

a predetermined amount
of treble droop

LXIX

Run an interconnecting cable
more than 4 to 6 feet long
between the output jack
on a preamp-control unit
to the input jack
on your power amplifier

LXX

If you wanted to tape record
music and voice to accompany a
showing of photographic
slides you would set up the
music on the changer or turntable,
adjust and mark maximum level,
then set up the microphone

LXXI

Fade in the music, bring
it down, fade in the voice

LXXII

Fade out the voice and bring up the music

Methods of Birth Control

> *"I'm rich, I'm smart, I can do what I want"*
> Margaret Sanger

I

Despite almost universal
failure to prevent conception
through administering internal
medicine, the same recipes used
in primitive societies
and in medieval Europe are used by
unsuspecting women

II

Herbal teas or other vegetable
concoctions are usually harmless, unlike
many common abortifacient
potions that can be deadly

III

marjoram
thyme
lavender
juniper   **may in fact be mild**
angelica   emmenagogues, stimulating
all-heal   the onset of menstruation
basil
hops
saffron
savory
celandine

IV

In many societies it was
believed that passivity during
intercourse would make a woman
less likely to conceive

V

Women engage in violent activities
immediately after intercourse in an
attempt to get the semen out of the
vagina

VI

Sneezing, after intercourse, was recommended
by the physicians of ancient Greece

VII

The Greek physician Aetios
knew the spermicidal properties
of vinegar, but instead of recommending
it to women as a douche,
he suggested applying it to the penis

VIII

In the 19th century
attempts to kill sperm
by bathing the penis in
some spermicidal lotion
were common

IX

Citrus fruit juices
can immobilize sperm
immediately

X

A pessary is a vaginal
suppository that will kill
spermatozoa and/or block their
path through the cervix

XI

The oldest of the extant Egyptian
papyri, the Petrie Papyrus of
1850 B.C., contains 3 perscriptions
for vaginal pessaries

XII

The use of crocodile dung in pessaries
was widespread

XIII

An Indian work of the first century B.C.
suggested rock soil dipped in oil, since
the oil would retard the mobility of sperm
and clog the cervix

XIV

Aristotle suggested either oil of cedar or olive oil

XV

The Ebers Papyrus of 1550 B.C.
prescribes a tampon made of lint
and saturated with a mixture of honey
and tips of acacia

XVI

The acacia shrub contains
gum arabic, the substance used
to produce lactic acid, the
spermicidal agent in most
modern contraceptive jellies

XVII

An anthropologist in Sumatra
was given a traditional contraceptive
suppository which turned out to contain
tannic acid

XVIII

In Africa women used plugs of chopped grass or cloth

XIX

Balls of bamboo tissue paper were used
by Japanese prostitutes

XX

Until the development of the rubber diaphragm
the sponge, first used by the Jews, was
the most efficient contraceptive

XXI

In a study done in New York
in 1930, Marie Kopp found that
women using sponges had a 50 per cent
success rate

XXII

Midwives in Java perform external
manipulations that cause the uterus
to tip, or become retroflexed,
thus preventing conception

XXIII

By the 18th century sheaths for
the penis were often given to
men by prostitutes

XXIV

In 1564 the Italian anatomist
Fallopius (discoverer of the "**Fallopian
tubes**") suggested a linen cloth
to fit the penis

XXV

In the late 18th century families
usually had eight children

XXVI

Increased public consciousness about
possible spread of venereal disease
from soldiers' and sailors' contacts
broke through official prudery to face
governmental action

XXVII

By 1919 the Army was spending a million dollars
on prophylactics

XXVIII

The development of vulcanized rubber
made the manufacture of condoms

easier and cheaper

XXIX

Although advertising contraceptives
was difficult because of censorship, douching
equipment had the advantage of having
multiple uses

XXX

There is probably not a druggist in the United States
who hasn't sold female syringes

XXXI

The Comstock Law of 1873
defined all contraceptive devices
as obscene

XXXII

On May 9, 1878
Dr. Sara Chase was
arrested and held for
$1500 bail at the
Tombs for having sold
two female syringes

XXXIII

After prominent figures like Arthur
Godfrey publicly announced their
own vasectomies, many individuals
abandoned the old tradition of secrecy
and described the personal advantages
of sterilization in the pages
of national publications

XXXIV

The clumsy insertion of a
diaphragm at an inopportune
moment

XXXV

Many adults are shocked when
they learn that boys and girls
of high school age ask questions
about contraceptives

XXXVI

"My friend says she knows she
won't get pregnant. Can she be sure?"

XXXVII

Although many bodily sensations,
including sexual ones, are pleasant,
there's more to life than sensual
enjoyment

XXXVIII

Petting and sexual intercourse mean
different things to different people

XXXIX

How can you say "no"
when you really mean "yes"?

XL

Abstinence appears to increase
the proportion of male sperm

XLI

Casanova is alleged to have
used a gold ball as a contraceptive,
placing it in the vagina to
block the sperm's passage

XLII

If Casanova managed not to
impregnate any of his girlfriends
(as he claimed), the most logical

explanation is that his frequent
ejaculations maintained his sperm
count at so low a level that
he was sterile in effect if not
in actuality

XLIII

Sexual abstinence ought to be
the means of avoiding not only
unwanted children but also
deleterious sexual excess

XLIV

The optimal time interval
between ejaculations to insure
maximum fertility is about
48 hours

XLV

Following the use of anti-
depressant drugs, sperm
production is accelerated and
fertility heightened

XLVI

He uses a condon
I use the Pill

XLVII

There may be live sperm
in the pre-coital fluid
that could survive in
favorable external vaginal mucus,
ultimately swimming ''upstream''
to the site of conception

XLVIII

Use of the diaphragm devolves
solely on the woman, and contraception
is no longer a joint venture
between a man and a woman
(as the condoms can be)

XLIX

Without abstinence, there is no natural family planning

L

Contraceptives such as the
Pill, diaphragm etc. are suitable
if the woman is able to assume
responsibility and isn't
subordinate to her husband

LI

If the man needs to be dominant
he may try to interfere with contraception

LII

A woman can
make a unilateral
i.e. private decision
to abandon use of the Pill
to achieve a desired pregnancy

LIII

A husband viewed his wife's
use of a diaphragm as a
demonstration not only of her love
for him but of her concern for
their shared physical relationship,
since it meant that *he*
didn't have to use a condom

LIV

There may be enough sperm
in the pre-ejaculatory fluids
to result in pregnancy

LV

Once you know on a day-to-day
basis whether or not a particular
act of intercourse is likely to lead
to conception, your "fertility
awareness" can then be used
either to postpone or avoid conception

LVI

A wife who feels "used"
during the sex act, may decide
to "get something" out of
the act of intercourse i.e. a baby
by "forgetting" to take the Pill

LVII

The obsessive-compulsive
personality type is an ideal candidate
for effective contraception

LVIII

The ability to maintain a prolonged relationship
reduces the number of exposures to new situations
when one may or may not be prepared with contraceptives

LIX

Despite its low batting
average as a successful
birth control method, for
religious reasons the rhythm
method is the only acceptable
one available to many people

LX

Judaism and Roman Catholicism
condemn the practice of *coitus
interruptus* but in Medieval Europe
its practice was common enough to
be frequently attacked as a "vice
against nature"

LXI

Withdraw penis before ejaculation
so that semen is deposited outside vagina

LXII

A religious observance of the calendar
or diligent recording of temperature
is no guarantee of protection
against unwanted pregnancy

LXIII

Simultaneous climaxes are necessary if conception
is to take place

LXIV

The transplant recipient became pregnant
and gave birth to a child
but the court ruled that the actual mother
was the donor of the ovary

LXV

Having sexual intercourse in a standing position
will prevent pregnancy

LXVI

Couples who have relied upon
this "method of contraception"
report it to be as successful

as French-kissing a water-moccasin

LXVII

There must be two acts of sexual
intercourse to produce twins, three for triplets

LXVIII

The Yellow Pages usually contain a list
of professional advisers you can contact
in confidence

LXIX

Louise Lacey is a woman, like many
other women, who recently decided to quit
taking the Pill

LXX

Farmers leave lights on in chicken
coops at night

LXXI

Owners of dress shops
who left naked wax
dummies in their windows
were convicted on the premise that
"bare dummies can cause
lustful thoughts"

LXXII

Like a river rising far off
and bearing down alluvium
from every shore, the notion
of birth control has picked up
philosophic debris on its long
course since Malthus

LXXIII

In some places
the sale of contraceptives
is carried on without
reticence

LXXIV

The instability of family life
and the disturbing increase of
divorces can be traced back
to the corrosive and shattering
effect of contraception

LXXV

By encouraging the "fit"
to procreate and discouraging
the "unfit," the world
would become a better place
in which to live

LXXVI

That any specific act
of intercourse in marriage may
be entered upon, even when
consciously nonprocreative, need
hardly be demonstrated

LXXVII

It would be a good
idea for you and your
wife to avoid
making love for about
five days

LXXVIII

The institution of syneisaktism
(spiritual marriage) whereby a
married couple live together but
conduct themselves as brother and sister
in the name of sexual asceticism

was a phenomenon of early Christianity
(and is not unknown today)

LXXIX

At the time of sexual enjoyment
press you finger on the forepart
of the testicle, turn your mind to
other things, and hold your breath

This book was set in Bem type at The Writer's Center,
Bethesda, Maryland.

Art Consultant: Kevin Osborn
Layout: Matthew Logan